ESSENTIAL GUIDE TO ERYTHEMA NODOSUM

Comprehensive Insights into Diagnosis, Management, and Treatment

DR. CASEY LOREN

DISCLAIMER

This book's content is only meant to be used for general informative purposes. Although the author has taken great care to ensure the content is accurate and thorough, no warranties or assurances on the information's accuracy, correctness, or reliability are provided. It is recommended that readers employ their own judgment and discretion when applying any material found in this book to their particular situation.

The information in this book is not intended to replace professional advice, nor is the author an expert in any of the subjects covered. It is recommended that readers consult with experienced professionals regarding any particular issues or concerns.

Any name that may be mentioned or referred in this book does not imply endorsement, recommendation, or relationship on the part of the author with any person, entity, good, website, or association. These references are made only for informational purposes and are not meant to be taken as recommendations or endorsements.

The information contained in this book may cause readers to suffer loss or damage, for which the author disclaims all obligation and accountability. The only people accountable for the decisions and actions taken by readers using the information presented are themselves.

Any names, characters, companies, locations, activities, occasions, and incidents referenced in this book are either made up or the result of the author's imagination. Any likeness to real people, living or dead, or to real things is entirely coincidental.

This book's content may change at any time, without prior notice, according to the author.

The onus is on the reader to verify whether there have been any updates or revisions.

The reader accepts the conditions of this disclaimer by reading this book. Please do not read this book or use its contents if you do not agree to these terms.

Table of Contents

CHAPTER 1

KNOWLEDGE OF ERYTHEMA NODOSUM

Overview and Definition of Erythema Nodosum

The inflammatory disease known as erythema nodosum (EN) is characterized by the abrupt appearance of painful red lumps or nodules under the skin, usually on the shins. It is a form of panniculitis, which indicates that the subcutaneous fat layer is inflamed. Several factors, such as infections, drugs, and systemic illnesses, can cause EN. The illness usually resolves on its own in a few weeks to months, but during flare-ups, it can be recurring and extremely uncomfortable.

Historical Context and Findings

The 19th century saw the first descriptions of Erythema nodosum. British dermatologist Robert Willan first used the term "erythema nodosum" in 1798. However, Hebra and other dermatologists did not characterize its clinical aspects more precisely until the middle of the 1800s. The understanding of EN has changed over time, leading to important discoveries about its pathophysiology and correlations with different underlying diseases.

The Epidemiology of Erythema Nodosum: Who Is at Risk?

Although EN can afflict people of any age, young adults between the ages of 20 and 40 are the most frequently affected. With a female-to-male ratio of about 3:1, women are impacted more often than men. In older adults and children under two, the disorder is quite uncommon. Geographically, spring and autumn are the seasons when EN is most common, as well as temperate climates.

Typical Indications and Symptoms

Tender, erythematous nodules, usually on the anterior regions of the lower legs, are the characteristic features of erythema nodosum. These nodules, which can occur in crops, typically have a diameter of 1 to 5 cm. Additional typical symptoms consist of:

- High temperature

- Malaise

Pain in the joints (arthralgia)

- Exhaustion

- Inflammation in the impacted regions

Like a bruise, the nodules frequently change color, ranging from a brilliant red to a reddish or brownish hue before disappearing.

Types and Arrangements

The two main categories for EN are acute and chronic:

1. **Acute Erythema Nodosum**: This type, which is the most prevalent, is typified by nodules that appear suddenly and go away in three to six weeks.

2. **Chronic Erythema Nodosum**: A less common type characterized by protracted periods of nodule recurrence.

The classification of EN can also take into account its correlation with other medical problems, drugs, or systemic illnesses (e.g., sarcoidosis, inflammatory bowel disease).

Pathophysiology: The Development of Erythema Nodosum

Although the precise pathophysiology of EN is unknown, immune-mediated responses are thought to be involved. To a range of antigens, it is regarded as a delayed hypersensitivity reaction. From a histopathological perspective, EN is distinguished by septal panniculitis in the absence of vasculitis, signifying inflammation restricted to the walls of fat rather than the lobules or blood vessels within fat.

Nodules are the result of a complicated interaction between immune cells, cytokines, and other inflammatory mediators throughout the inflammatory process.

Risk Elements and Contributing Factors

Several circumstances and characteristics that make someone more likely to get EN:

- TB, fungal, and streptococcal infections are among the **Infections**.

- **Medications**: oral contraceptives, sulfonamides, and certain antibiotics.

- **Systemic Diseases**: ulcerative colitis, sarcoidosis, and several types of cancer are inflammatory bowel diseases.

- **Pregnancy**: Changes in hormones can result in EN.

Genetic Predisposition: A family history of autoimmune illnesses connected to EN or similar disorders.

Differential Diagnosis: Excluded Conditions

Accurate diagnosis and treatment of EN depend on its ability to be distinguished from other illnesses with similar symptoms. Among the conditions to take into account for the differential diagnosis are:

Cellulitis: A less nodular and more diffuse kind of bacterial skin infection.

Erythema induratum: An additional type of panniculitis that is frequently connected to tuberculosis.

- **Nodular vasculitis**: A condition where blood vessels in subcutaneous tissue become inflamed.

- **Liposarcoma**: A very uncommon kind of cancer that can appear as nodules under the skin.

Issues and the Outlook

In most cases, EN is a self-limiting illness with a favorable prognosis. In a matter of weeks to months, the majority of instances end without causing long-term harm. But difficulties can occur, especially if the fundamental problem is ignored:

Persistent or recurring episodes: Particularly in cases with long-term EN.

- **Hyperpigmentation**: Skin pigmentation changes following an inflammatory response.

- **Arthritis**: In certain situations, joint pain might become chronic.

The Value of Early Identification

It is crucial to identify EN early for several reasons:

- **Symptom Management**: Prompt action can reduce symptoms and enhance life expectancy.

Determination of Underlying Causes: Early diagnosis and treatment of underlying illnesses, such as infections or systemic diseases, can assist to discover and stop more complications.

- **Preventing Recurrences**: Recurrent episodes can be avoided by being aware of and in control of triggers.

To sum up, erythema nodosum is a complex illness with a wide range of underlying causes and comorbidities. Improving patient outcomes and quality of life requires proper understanding, early discovery, and care.

CHAPTER 2

REASONS AND INITIATORS

Erythema Nodosum Causes and Triggers

An inflammatory skin ailment called erythema nodosum (EN) is typified by sensitive, red nodules that are typically found on the shins. Comprehending the diverse origins and initiators of EN is imperative for precise diagnosis, suitable handling, and tackling fundamental elements that contribute to the ailment. Let's examine each in more detail:

Contagious Origins

A prominent cause of EN is infection; bacterial and viral pathogens are thought to play a role in the disease's development. One well-known infectious cause of EN is streptococcal infections, such as streptococcal pharyngitis (strep throat). EN can also be brought on by other bacterial infections such as Yersinia, Mycoplasma, and TB, as well as viral infections such as Epstein-Barr virus (EBV) and herpes simplex virus (HSV).

Medication-Induced Erythema Nodosum

As a hypersensitive reaction, EN has been linked to specific drugs. These medications include non-steroidal anti-inflammatory drugs (NSAIDs), oral contraceptives, some anticonvulsants, and antibiotics such as sulfonamides, penicillins, and tetracyclines. The key to treating drug-induced EN is figuring out whatever medicine is causing it and stopping it.

Systemic and Autoimmune Disorders

EN may be a sign of underlying immunological dysregulation and be linked to several autoimmune and systemic illnesses.

Sarcoidosis, Behçet's illness, rheumatoid arthritis, and inflammatory bowel disease (Crohn's disease, ulcerative colitis) are among the conditions that are frequently associated with EN. In these situations, addressing the autoimmune or systemic disease that underlies EN is essential.

Hormonal Factors

EN development may be influenced by hormonal imbalances and fluctuations, especially in women. The use of oral contraceptives, pregnancy, and hormone treatments can all cause EN episodes because of their effects on inflammatory pathways and immunological responses. Women with recurrent EN linked to hormonal issues may require hormonal examination and treatment.

Hereditary Propensity

Given that EN can manifest itself more frequently in some people or families, there may be a hereditary predisposition to acquiring the condition. The pathophysiology of EN may be influenced by genetic variables that affect inflammatory responses, immune system function, and susceptibility to infections or hypersensitivity reactions. It will take more investigation to identify particular genetic markers linked to EN.

Environmental Stressors

For those who are sensitive, environmental variables like cold temperature, trauma, and exposure to specific chemicals or allergens can cause EN. Vasoconstriction and alterations in immunological responses can cause cold-induced EN, also referred to as "winter EN," to happen during the colder months. EN flare-ups can be avoided by avoiding triggers and shielding the skin from environmental aggressors.

Typical Irritants and Allergens

Cosmetics, detergents, textiles, topical treatments, and other allergens and irritants can cause hypersensitive reactions that result in EN. Skin lesions resembling ENs can be a symptom of contact dermatitis or allergies to particular compounds. The key to treating EN brought on by these causes is recognizing and avoiding allergens and irritants.

Erythema Nodosum and Lifestyle Factors

Smoking, stress, and inadequate diet are a few lifestyle variables that can affect the intensity and susceptibility of EN. For those with EN, quitting smoking and embracing a healthy lifestyle that includes stress reduction and a balanced diet can help lower inflammation and enhance general skin health.

Idiopathic Nodosum Erythematosus

Idiopathic EN is a type of EN that can occasionally occur with no known reason. The lack of a clear underlying cause or specific trigger makes it difficult to diagnose and treat idiopathic EN. To rule out other possible causes, a comprehensive evaluation that includes a complete medical history, physical examination, and laboratory tests may be required.

Examples and Case Studies

Insights into the various origins and triggers of EN can be gained from case studies and clinical experiences. An example of an infectious cause of EN in a young adult is a case of streptococcal pharyngitis. A further instance of a drug-induced hypersensitive reaction to a sulfa antibiotic highlights the part that drugs play in the development of EN. The significance of a comprehensive assessment and customized management approaches in EN circumstances is emphasized by real-world instances.

To summarise, there are several potential causes and triggers for Erythema Nodosum, including drugs, autoimmune illnesses, infections, hormonal variables, environmental triggers, allergens, lifestyle factors, genetic predispositions, and idiopathic factors. Effective management of EN and the avoidance of recurring flare-ups depend on the identification and treatment of these underlying causes.

CHAPTER 3

IDENTIFICATION AND ASSESSMENT

Preliminary Clinical Assessment

To properly diagnose erythema nodosum, a patient's medical history, present symptoms, and physical examination must all be thoroughly evaluated. Finding possible triggers or underlying disorders that might be influencing the development of erythema nodosum depends on the results of this evaluation.

Comprehensive Health Background

To fully comprehend the patient's overall health, past medical issues, medication history, exposure to infections, travel history, and any recent illnesses or injuries, a thorough medical history must be taken. This data aids in determining possible reasons or connections to erythema nodosum.

Methods of Physical Examination

Healthcare professionals search for distinctive erythema nodosum symptoms during the physical examination, such as sensitive, red, elevated nodules on the skin, usually on the shins. Additionally, they look for indications of underlying diseases like joint discomfort, fever, or stomach problems that could be connected to erythema nodosum.

Biomarkers and Blood Tests

Blood tests can be used to diagnose autoimmune illnesses, inflammatory problems, or infections that may be linked to erythema nodosum. Infections that may include rheumatoid arthritis, sarcoidosis, or streptococcal infections are examples of these. The antinuclear antibody (ANA) test, C-reactive protein (CRP), erythrocyte sedimentation rate (ESR), complete blood count (CBC), and certain infection markers are examples of common blood tests.

Imaging Studies (ultrasonography, CT scans, etc.)

To find any underlying abnormalities, such as joint effusions, lung infiltrates, or enlarged lymph nodes, imaging procedures like X-rays and ultrasounds may be carried out. These studies can aid in determining potential causes of erythema nodosum.

Histopathology and Biopsy

To confirm the diagnosis of erythema nodosum, a skin biopsy might be suggested. In a biopsy, a tiny sample of skin tissue is removed, and it is analyzed under a microscope (histopathology) to search for signs of panniculitis, or inflammation in the fatty tissue beneath the skin, which are typical characteristics of erythema nodosum.

Process of Differential Diagnosis

Erythema multiforme, cellulitis, vasculitis, and insect bites are among the skin disorders that must be differentiated from one another to make a differential diagnosis of erythema nodosum. The patient's clinical presentation, medical history, and findings of any diagnostic tests must all be carefully taken into account during this process.

The Function of Expert Consultations

Consultations with specialists may be required, depending on the symptoms that are related or the probable underlying reason. This could include, among others, gastroenterologists, rheumatologists, dermatologists, and experts in infectious diseases. Care that is collaborative guarantees a careful assessment and suitable handling.

Analysing Test Outcomes

To determine the underlying cause of erythema nodosum, test data from imaging investigations, blood tests, and biopsy reports must be analyzed. Anomalies in particular biomarkers or imaging results can offer important hints to direct more research and therapy.

Verifying the Medical Diagnose

Integrating data from the initial assessment, medical history, physical examination, laboratory testing, imaging studies, and histopathological findings is necessary for diagnosis confirmation. Once other possible causes have been checked out and diagnostic signs are present, erythema nodosum is definitively diagnosed.

In general, erythema nodosum and its underlying causes or linked disorders must be appropriately diagnosed by a methodical and comprehensive approach to testing and diagnosis. Patients with this illness receive comprehensive care and optimal management through collaboration between healthcare providers and specialists.

CHAPTER 4

THERAPY AND ADMINISTRATION

Synopsis of Therapy Objectives

The main objectives of erythema nodosum (EN) management are symptom relief, inflammation reduction, and, if known, addressing underlying causes. A variety of drugs, lifestyle changes, and individualized supportive therapies are frequently used in treatment plans.

Drugs: Corticosteroids, NSAIDs, and Other

NSAIDs (Nonsteroidal Anti-Inflammatory Drugs): These are frequently prescribed to treat EN-related pain and inflammation.

Corticosteroids: To reduce inflammation and suppress the immune response in more severe situations or when NSAIDs are not enough, a prescription for corticosteroids may be given.

Other Medications: Other medications like potassium iodide, colchicine, or immunosuppressive treatments like methotrexate may be taken into consideration, depending on the underlying reason or particular symptoms.

Treatments Inhibiting Immunity

Immunosuppressive treatments such as cyclosporine, azathioprine, or methotrexate may be recommended for resistant or severe instances of EN to suppress the immune system and lessen inflammation.

Antibiotic Therapies for Viral Infections

It could be required to administer the proper antibiotic medication directed against the particular pathogen if EN is brought on by an underlying illness.

Modifications to Lifestyle

Rest: To encourage healing and lessen stress on the body, getting enough sleep is essential during acute flare-ups.

Avoiding Triggers: Recurrences can be avoided by recognizing and staying away from potential triggers like specific drugs, illnesses, or environmental conditions.

Dietary Guidelines

Although there are no particular dietary recommendations for EN, the immune system and general health can be supported by eating a well-balanced, nutrient-rich diet.

Techniques for Pain Management

Topical Treatments: Localised pain treatment can be achieved with creams or ointments that contain analgesic or anti-inflammatory drugs.

Oral Pain Medications: Prescription or over-the-counter painkillers may be suggested, depending on the degree of pain.

Exercise and Physical Therapy

Gentle Exercise: Walking and swimming are examples of low-impact exercises that can help preserve mobility and enhance circulation without aggravating symptoms.

Physical Therapy: Physical therapy can help with strengthening and rehabilitation when EN impairs joint function or mobility.

Observation and Aftercare

It is crucial to schedule routine follow-up visits with medical professionals to assess treatment outcomes, track advancements, and address any emerging symptoms or concerns.

Tailored Care Programmes

A customized treatment plan may be necessary for each EN patient, taking into account variables including the underlying cause, degree of symptoms, medical background, and reaction to previous treatments. Plans for personalized treatment make sure that interventions are customized to fit individual needs and maximize results.

By incorporating these elements into a thorough treatment plan, medical professionals can better manage EN and enhance the quality of life for their patients.

CHAPTER 5

LIVING WITH NODOSUM ERYTHEMATOSUS

Modifications to Daily Life

To properly control symptoms, living with Erythema Nodosum necessitates significant adaptations to everyday routine. These modifications could consist of:

Symptom Monitoring: Keep a record of any new symptoms that may appear, pain thresholds, and flare-ups.

- **Balanced Diet:** Maintain a healthy, well-balanced diet to boost your general well-being and immune system.

- **Regular Exercise:** Take part in low-impact activities like yoga, swimming, or walking that won't make inflammation worse.

- **Adequate Rest:** To promote stress relief and bodily healing, make sure you receive adequate sleep every night.

- **Avoiding Triggers:** Recognise and stay away from things like particular drugs or environments that could exacerbate your symptoms.

Handling Remissions and Flares

Remissions and flare-ups are frequent in Erythema Nodosum cases. These are some methods to deal with them:

- **Medication Compliance:** To control pain and inflammation during flare-ups, take prescription drugs as advised by your doctor.

Monitoring: Keep an eye on the things that cause flare-ups and, if you can, take preventative action.

- **Seeking Immediate Medical Attention**: See your doctor right away if you suffer a significant flare-up or develop any new symptoms.

Effects on Emotion and Psychology

Living with a long-term medical illness such as Erythema Nodosum can lead to psychological and emotional consequences. It's critical to:

- **Seek Support:** To deal with emotional difficulties, think about speaking with a therapist or attending a support group.

- **Practice tension Management:** To lessen tension and anxiety, try deep breathing exercises, meditation, or engaging in hobbies.

Remain Informed: Gain knowledge about the illness to help you feel more in charge and empowered.

Coping Mechanisms and Support Networks

Having a solid support network and learning coping mechanisms can help:

- **Mindfulness:** To stay in the present and lessen worry about the future, engage in mindfulness exercises.

- **Support Groups:** Make connections with people going through similar struggles by joining online or live support groups.

- **Open Communication:** Share your wants and worries honestly and openly with your family, friends, and healthcare staff.

Self-Care Advice and Methods

Taking care of oneself is essential for treating erythema nodosum:

- **Skin Care:** To avoid irritation and infections, keep your skin moisturized and clean.

Discomfort Management: As directed by your healthcare practitioner, apply heat packs or cold compresses to reduce discomfort and inflammation.

- **Healthy Habits:** To promote general health, give up drinking, stop smoking, and keep a healthy weight.

Navigating Work and Social Life

Adjustments may be necessary to manage job and social life when dealing with Erythema Nodosum:

- **Flexible Work Arrangements:** If symptoms require it, take into account modifying your schedule or making accommodations.

-    **Educating Others:** To foster understanding and support, educate friends and coworkers about your condition.

Setting Boundaries: Develop the ability to say no when it's important to take care of yourself and control your energy levels.

Handling Mobility Concerns

There may be changes in mobility during flare-ups. Think about:

- **Assistive equipment:** If you have limited mobility, use assistive equipment like walkers or canes.

- **Physical Therapy:** To increase strength and mobility, perform physical therapy exercises.

Home Modifications: Adjust your home as needed to improve accessibility when your mobility is restricted.

Interaction with Friends and Family

The secret to getting support from loved ones is having open communication:

- **Educate Loved Ones:** Make sure your friends and family are aware of your condition, its effects, and how they can help.

Express Needs: Clearly state what you need and what you can't do so that others can help you.

- **Gratitude:** Show your appreciation for their help and understanding to strengthen your bonds with them.

Establishing a Network of Support

Having a robust support system is crucial:

- **Healthcare Team:** For all-encompassing care, establish a cooperative connection with your healthcare team.

- **Family and Friends:** For both practical and emotional assistance, rely on your friends and family.

- **Support Groups:** Make connections with people who have experienced similar things by joining online or local support groups.

Extended Prognosis

Keeping an optimistic long-term perspective entails:

Regular Check-ups: Continue to follow up on screenings and follow-up appointments to keep an eye on your health.

Adapting as Needed: Have an open mind and be prepared to modify your treatment strategy and way of life as circumstances demand.

- **Hope and Positivity:** Keep your eyes on your progress and hold onto your optimism for more developments in treatment alternatives in the future.

Erythema Nodosum necessitates a multifaceted lifestyle that takes into account social, emotional, and physical facets. You can enhance your quality of life and prospects by taking proactive measures to manage your condition, getting help when needed, and making the required modifications.

CHAPTER 6

ERYTHEMA NODOSUM IN PARTICULAR GROUPS

Youngsters and Teenagers

The special issues associated with erythema nodosum (EN) in children and adolescents stem from the possibility of misdiagnosis and its impact on growth and development. In this group, the diagnosis can be more difficult because a variety of illnesses, such as infections or inflammatory disorders, can present with identical symptoms. Typically, treatment includes treating the underlying cause in addition to controlling symptoms like pain and inflammation. Ensuring optimal outcomes throughout treatment necessitates close monitoring of growth and development.

Women Who Are Expecting

Because there may be dangers to the mother and fetus, managing erythema nodosum in pregnant women needs to be done with great care. Careful consideration must be given to treatment alternatives to minimize side effects and successfully manage symptoms. Because non-steroidal anti-inflammatory medicines (NSAIDs) have the potential to impact fetal development, they are typically avoided. Throughout the pregnancy, close observation by medical professionals is necessary to guarantee the best possible outcome for the mother and child.

Senior Citizens

Comorbidities and decreased tolerance to specific drugs are two additional obstacles that elderly people with erythema nodosum may face. The underlying cause of EN in this population needs to be carefully assessed because it may be connected to age-related illnesses such as infections or cancers. Treatment plans must be customized for each patient, taking into consideration any possible drug interactions and adverse effects on senior citizens.

Individuals with Prior Medical Conditions

Erythema nodosum may be more likely to occur in patients with pre-existing diseases such as autoimmune illnesses or chronic infections. In these situations, managing the patient generally entails treating both the symptoms of EN and the underlying cause. For patients with complicated medical histories, close coordination among specialists is essential to provide complete care and the best possible results.

Erythema Nodosum Gender Differences

Males and females may exhibit erythema nodosum differently, even though it can affect people of either gender. For instance, one gender may be more affected than the other by specific diseases or drugs that are more frequently linked to EN. Healthcare professionals can better personalize diagnosis and treatment plans based on gender-specific risk factors and considerations by being aware of these variances.

Differences by Region and Ethnicity

Geographic and ethnic variations are seen in the prevalence and related circumstances of erythema nodosum. Because of endemic infections or other environmental variables, some regions may have a greater prevalence of EN. Susceptibility to particular triggers or underlying conditions that can cause EN can also be influenced by ethnicity. Accurate diagnosis and population-specific therapy techniques depend on taking these variances into account.

Physically Active People and Athletes**

Managing erythema nodosum can present special difficulties for athletes and physically active people, especially if the condition interferes with their capacity to play sports or exercise. To prevent complications or exacerbations, careful monitoring of symptoms and modifications to activity levels may be required during treatment. Working together with specialists in sports medicine can help maximize care for this population.

Professional Risks and Things to Think About

Erythema nodosum may be more common in certain activities or exposures, such as those involving possible allergens or irritants. When diagnosing EN, occupational history should be taken into account to determine potential factors or triggers. It may be advised to implement occupational health precautions, such as protective gear and environmental controls, to stop the symptoms from getting worse or from returning.

In Particular, Immunocompromised Patients Should Take into Account

When treating erythema nodosum, individuals who are immunocompromised—such as those with HIV/AIDS or receiving immunosuppressive therapy—need to be treated with extra caution. Their immunocompromised state or additional opportunistic infections could be the underlying reason. Treatment plans must strike a compromise between reducing the chance of complications or worsening the underlying immunodeficiency and managing the symptoms of EN.

Case Studies Illustrating Various Populations:

Case studies showcasing erythema nodosum in various demographics can offer important insights into difficulties with diagnosis, methods of therapy, and results. Based on factors such as age, gender, ethnicity, and comorbidities, these case studies can illustrate differences in presentation, underlying causes, and response to therapy. Real-world case analysis can enhance clinical judgment and enhance patient treatment for a range of EN-affected groups.

CHAPTER 7

INVESTIGATIONS AND NEW TREATMENTS

Present Research Patterns

Currently, research on Erythema Nodosum (EN) is concentrated in a few important areas. Investigating the underlying causes of EN, including autoimmune, hypersensitivity, and viral factors, is one popular trend. Researchers are also looking into how genetic predisposition and immune system malfunction contribute to the development of EN. Furthermore, the relationship between EN and other systemic illnesses like sarcoidosis and inflammatory bowel disease is a subject of increasing attention.

Current Clinical Trial Results

Numerous therapeutic approaches for EN, such as corticosteroids, immunomodulatory medications, and nonsteroidal anti-inflammatory medicines (NSAIDs), have been investigated in recent clinical trials. The results of these trials have aided in the improvement of EN patient outcomes and treatment regimens. Furthermore, research has demonstrated the significance of timely diagnosis and focused treatment approaches in mitigating the severity and recurrence of disease.

Progress in Genetics and Immunology

Developments in genetics and immunology have illuminated the pathophysiology of EN. Immunological investigations have shown that patients with EN have anomalies in T cell activity and cytokine production. Specific gene variants linked to an increased chance of developing EN have been found through genetic investigations, offering important new information about disease susceptibility and possible treatment options.

Innovative Therapeutic Strategies

Targeted biologics like interleukin-1 antagonists and TNF-alpha inhibitors are examples of novel therapy strategies for EN. In refractory cases of EN, these medicines have demonstrated encouraging success in terms of lowering inflammation and enhancing clinical outcomes. Patients with EN now have more alternatives thanks to immune modulators, phototherapy, and topical treatments, among other cutting-edge medications.

Biotechnology's Place in Treatment

The creation of cutting-edge EN therapy alternatives heavily relies on biotechnology.

Produced by biotechnological techniques, biologic medications target certain critical components in the inflammatory cascade, allowing for more targeted and efficient therapy. Additionally, biotechnology makes personalized medicine possible by customizing treatment plans according to the unique characteristics of each patient and the disease profile.

Complementary and Alternative Health

Acupuncture, herbal supplements, and mind-body therapies are examples of integrative and alternative medicine methods that are being investigated as supplementary treatments for EN. Even though further studies are required to determine their effectiveness, some individuals might benefit from these strategies when included in an all-encompassing therapy strategy. Integrative treatment is centered on attending to patients' needs holistically, which includes their mental, emotional, and spiritual health.

Prospects for Erythema Nodosum Research in the Future

The development of tailored immunotherapies, the identification of novel biomarkers for disease activity and prognosis, and the use of precision medicine techniques to optimize treatment algorithms are some of the future research directions in EN. Multidisciplinary teams working together are crucial to expanding our knowledge of EN and enhancing patient outcomes.

Involvement of Patients in Research

Patient involvement in research is essential to expanding our understanding of EN and enhancing patient care. Research validity and relevance are increased through patient participation in clinical trials, patient-reported outcome metrics, and shared decision-making processes. Educating and advocating for patients' rights also raises awareness and makes it easier for the community to support EN research projects.

Ethical Issues in Research on Erythema Nodosum

Informed permission, fair access to research opportunities, patient privacy and confidentiality, and appropriate sharing of research findings are among the ethical factors that EN researchers must take into account. Throughout the research process, researchers and healthcare professionals must respect ethical norms and give patients' well-being a top priority.

Connecting Clinical Practice and Research

Translating scientific findings into practical applications requires a bridge between research and clinical practice. Evidence-based practice in EN management is promoted and knowledge transfer is facilitated through collaborative networks, continuing education initiatives, and clinical recommendations. Applying research findings to improve patient care and outcomes is a critical job for clinicians.

By focusing on these crucial areas in EN research and developing treatments, we may increase our knowledge of the illness, expand our therapeutic options, and eventually raise the standard of living for Erythema Nodosum patients.

CHAPTER 8

KEEPING ERYTHEMA NODOSUM AT BAY

Determining and Steering Clear of Triggers:

Skin irritation known as erythema nodosum is frequently brought on by several different sources. The key to stopping its incidence or recurrence is recognizing and avoiding these triggers. Certain medications, including antibiotics, oral contraceptives, and nonsteroidal anti-inflammatory drugs (NSAIDs), are frequently identified as triggers. Erythema nodosum can also be brought on by illnesses like tuberculosis, fungal infections, or streptococcal infections. Other potential triggers include environmental factors including exposure to cold temperatures or allergens, as well as autoimmune illnesses like sarcoidosis or inflammatory bowel disease.

Medications for Prevention:

Healthcare practitioners may provide preventive drugs in some instances to lower the incidence of erythema nodosum. These drugs may be immunosuppressants, such as corticosteroids, which reduce inflammation, or they may be designed to treat particular underlying illnesses, including autoimmune diseases. When using preventive medication, it's critical to pay great attention to the doctor's instructions because these drugs have potential adverse effects and need to be monitored frequently.

Immunisation and Vaccination Techniques

Erythema nodosum can be brought on by a few illnesses, including tuberculosis and streptococcal infections. Immunization and vaccination programs can lessen the chance of contracting erythema nodosum by preventing certain illnesses. Infections with streptococci or tuberculosis may require vaccinations; this recommendation is dependent on a person's medical history and risk factors.

Well-Being Lifestyle Options

Preventing erythema nodosum can also be achieved by leading a healthy lifestyle. This includes getting enough sleep, exercising frequently, maintaining a healthy diet high in fruits, vegetables, and whole grains, and abstaining from tobacco and excessive alcohol use. These lifestyle decisions lessen the chance of developing specific infections and inflammatory diseases while also promoting the health of the immune system as a whole.

Management Strategies for Stress

Erythema nodosum and other inflammatory diseases might get worse under stress. Reducing stress can be achieved by putting stress management practices into practice, such as mindfulness meditation, yoga, deep breathing exercises, and counseling or support group participation. Effective stress management can help stop flare-ups or the worsening of erythema nodosum symptoms.

Consistent Health Examinations

For people who have underlying medical disorders that may cause erythema nodosum or who are at risk of developing it, routine medical check-ups are crucial. These examinations give medical practitioners the chance to keep an eye on patients' general health, successfully treat underlying illnesses, and alter prescriptions or preventive measures as needed.

Initial Intervention Techniques

For erythema nodosum to be managed, early intervention is essential. Early symptom recognition and timely medical intervention are key to avoiding problems and achieving better results. Medication to control discomfort, lower inflammation, or treat underlying issues causing erythema nodosum are some possible treatment options.

Programmes for Education and Awareness

Programs for raising awareness and promoting education are essential for preventing erythema nodosum. The purpose of these programs is to inform people about the illness, including its symptoms, triggers, and management techniques. Raising awareness among medical professionals, patients, and the general public can help those with erythema nodosum get better care, experience earlier detection, and live better lives.

Public Health Initiatives' Role

A larger-scale approach to treating erythema nodosum depends on public health programs. Campaigns for vaccinations against illnesses that might cause erythema nodosum, encouragement of good lifestyle choices, public health campaigns to increase awareness, and funding for research into preventive and therapeutic measures are a few examples of these endeavors.

Creating a Customised Prevention Strategy

Individuals who have a history of erythema nodosum or who are at risk for the condition must develop a customized preventive plan. Together with healthcare professionals, this plan should be created. It may include tactics like recognizing and avoiding triggers, leading a healthy lifestyle, getting recommended vaccinations, effectively managing stress, scheduling routine check-ups, and putting early intervention strategies in place.

People and healthcare professionals may collaborate to successfully avoid erythema nodosum and enhance overall health outcomes for those who are impacted by this condition by thoroughly addressing these important factors.

CHAPTER 9

PATIENT NARRATIVES AND CASE STUDIES

* Detailed Case Studies with Analysis:

Case studies are a great way to learn about the subtle differences between Erythema Nodosum and other conditions. They offer a thorough understanding of the symptoms, diagnosis, treatment modalities, and results of the patient. By examining these cases, patterns, triggers, and patient-specific differences in responsiveness to treatment can be identified.

Erythema Nodosum Success tales

These tales illustrate cases in which patients have successfully treated EN. These narratives frequently highlight the importance of early diagnosis, suitable treatment regimens, lifestyle adjustments, and routine follow-ups. They can demonstrate the value of proactive management and provide people with EN hope and optimism.

Difficulties and Difficulties Faced by Patients

Individuals with EN face a variety of difficulties, such as incorrect diagnosis, postponed treatment, frequent flare-ups, discomfort in the body, and psychological distress. Healthcare professionals must comprehend these difficulties to provide complete support and modify treatment plans appropriately.

Personal Narratives of Coping with Erythema Nodosum

Personal narratives offer firsthand perspectives on the day-to-day challenges, difficulties, and coping strategies of people with EN. These accounts provide insight into how EN affects relationships, employment, mental health, and overall quality of life.

Lessons Learned from Patient Experiences

Healthcare professionals may learn a lot from patient experiences, such as the value of prompt diagnosis, customized treatment regimens, patient education, emotional support, and all-encompassing care. Gaining knowledge from these events improves patient outcomes and clinical practice.

Impact of Various Treatments on Patients: The degree, underlying causes, and reactions of patients determine how different EN treatment modalities are used. Optimizing results and improving treatment algorithms are made possible by evaluating the effects of therapies including corticosteroids, immunomodulators, nonsteroidal anti-inflammatory medications (NSAIDs), and lifestyle changes.

Many Results in Erythema Nodosum Management: The results of managing EN might vary from total symptom relief to persistent or recurrent symptoms. Comorbidities, patient-specific characteristics, treatment adherence, and illness severity are all factors that affect the results. Long-term monitoring and treatment planning are guided by the analysis of various outcomes.

Psychological and Social Aspects

EN's physical symptoms frequently converge with social and psychological elements, resulting in relational difficulties, emotional distress, and issues with body image. Enhancing overall well-being and treatment adherence can be achieved by addressing these characteristics through psychological support, counseling, and patient advocacy.

Inspiring Stories of Overcoming Adversity

Despite EN hurdles, inspirational stories emphasize resiliency, tenacity, and successful outcomes. These narratives honor the successes of patients, the work of advocates, the generosity of the community, and the ability of optimism to manage long-term illnesses like EN.

Contributions from Healthcare Providers

Healthcare providers play a vital role in EN management through correct diagnosis, evidence-based treatment, patient education, multidisciplinary teamwork, and continuous support. Sharing insights, best practices, and collaborative efforts across providers improves patient care and outcomes.

Through a thorough examination of these facets, the indispensable Erythema Nodosum guide may provide a comprehensive grasp of the ailment, its handling, and the patient experience, which will be advantageous to both medical professionals and those impacted by EN.

CHAPTER 10

MATERIALS AND ASSISTANCE

Assets Related to Insurance and Financial Assistance

- **Financial support Programmes:** Look into programs run by the government, charitable organizations, and pharmaceutical companies that may provide medicine discounts or financial support.

- **Health Insurance Coverage:** Recognise what is and is not covered by your insurance policy for prescription drugs, therapies, medical visits, and hospital stays for erythema nodosum. For clarification on the specifics of your plan, get in touch with your insurer.

- **Medical Bills Management:** Manage your insurance claims, bills, and medical spending.

Make use of financial resources like medical savings accounts or healthcare providers' payment plans.

Learning Resources and Workshops

- **Online Resources:** For the most recent information and research findings, visit reliable websites, medical journals, and forums devoted to erythema nodosum.

- **Workshops and Seminars:** Learn about managing symptoms, treatment options, and lifestyle modifications by attending workshops hosted by healthcare organizations or patient advocacy groups.

Creating a Plan of Care

- **Medical Team Collaboration:** To create an all-encompassing care plan, collaborate closely with rheumatologists, dermatologists, and primary care physicians.

- **Treatment Objectives:** Set specific objectives to control symptoms, enhance life quality, and stop flare-ups.

- **Medication Schedule:** Adhere to recommended dosage regimens and assess how well they are managing erythema nodosum.

Workplace and Legal Considerations

- **Disability Benefits:** If your erythema nodosum considerably affects your capacity to work, consider your eligibility for disability benefits.

Workplace Accommodations: Discuss possible accommodations for your health needs, such as ergonomic modifications or flexible work schedules, with your employer.

Moving Through Health Systems

- **Healthcare Advocacy:** Assign a reliable advocate or healthcare proxy to help with appointment scheduling, interacting with medical experts, and navigating complicated healthcare systems.

- **Second Opinions:** To guarantee correct diagnosis and suitable treatment strategies, get second opinions from experts.

Patient Rights and Advocacy

- **Know Your Rights:** Educate yourself on the rights of patients, such as the right to privacy, informed consent, and access to medical records.

- **Advocacy Groups:** To keep educated, connect with support systems, and push for better healthcare regulations, join patient advocacy groups devoted to erythema nodosum.

Tips for Self-Care

- **Healthy Lifestyle:** Make rest a priority, exercise frequently, and keep a balanced diet.

- **Skin Care:** To control erythema nodosum-related skin problems, adhere to your dermatologist's suggested skincare regimen.

- **Stress Management:** To manage the emotional effects of the illness, engage in stress-reduction practices like yoga, meditation, or counseling.

Mechanisms of Coping

- **Support Networks:** Make connections with loved ones, friends, and support groups to exchange coping mechanisms, seek and provide emotional support, and share experiences.

- **Therapeutic Activities:** Take up creative endeavors, hobbies, or mindfulness exercises to build resilience and emotional well-being.

- **Professional Counselling:** To address the emotional difficulties, anxiety, or sadness that come with having a chronic illness, think about attending counseling or therapy sessions.

Resources for carers

- **Carer Support Groups:** To address carer stress, burnout, and emotional well-being, encourage carers to attend support groups or counseling sessions.

- **Respite Care:** Examine your alternatives for temporary relief and self-care time for carers through respite care services.

To effectively manage erythema nodosum, each of these factors is essential for meeting practical, emotional, and economic needs as well as fostering general well-being.